# Exercise Equivalents of Foods

**A Practical Guide for the Overweight**

## Frank Konishi

SOUTHERN ILLINOIS UNIVERSITY PRESS
Carbondale and Edwardsville

Feffer & Simons, Inc.
London and Amsterdam

**Library of Congress Cataloging in Publication Data**

Konishi, Frank
  Exercise equivalents of foods.


  (Arcturus books, AB 131)
  1.  Exercise — Physiological  effect.  2.  Reducing  exercises.  3.  Food —
Caloric content — Tables.   I.   Title.
RA781.6.K66   1975          613.7′1          75–1294
ISBN 0–8093–0736–7 pbk.

Copyright © 1973 by Southern Illinois University Press
All rights reserved
Arcturus Books Edition August 1975
Second printing November 1976
This edition printed by offset lithography in the
  United States of America
Designed by Gary Gore

# Contents

# List of Tables

# Introduction

The significance of proper exercise as an integral part of a weight reducing program is frequently minimized. This is surprising since the calories expended in physical activity may comprise the greatest portion of the total daily energy expenditure. For example, if an individual is engaged in hard physical labor, the total calories expended can exceed 6,000 Cal per day.* This would represent an expenditure of 3,200 Cal more than the total calories recommended for the average male adult living in the United States. Comparable intakes by a sedentary individual obviously would result in an accumulation of body fat and subsequent obesity.

It is apparent then, that exercise should be a major factor to consider in preventing or treating obesity. The prevalence of obesity in the United States, however, would indicate that many individuals fail to appreciate the value of adequate exercise. This may be due partially to an unawareness of the quantitative value of the activity in terms of calories expended. This is not surprising inasmuch as complete tables of the caloric costs of various activities are not readily available, or if available, subject to misinterpretation.

One method of relating exercise and calories in food would be to develop tables of food energy values in terms of energy equivalents of various activities.[1] The energy or caloric value of a specific food would be reported in terms of equivalents of time spent in certain activities. The time values for a specific food, then, would vary inversely as the energy cost of the activity increases. This book presents data relating exercise to calories in food by listing the exercise equivalents of over six hundred common

*A calorie is defined as the amount of heat required at a pressure of one atmosphere to raise the temperature of one gram of water one degree centigrade. A kilocalorie (kcal) or large calorie (Cal), equals one thousand calories, and is defined as the amount of heat required to raise one kilogram of water one degree centigrade. It is used as a unit in expressing the heat-producing or energy-producing value of food. The specific caloric values in this book and in most diet guides are actually kilocalories, and will be referred to by the scientific abbreviation Cal.

# Introduction

foods using the average energy cost for walking, bicycling, stepping, swimming, and jogging. It is designed to furnish practical information for use by parents, teachers, dietitians, physicians, or any other individual concerned with the prevention and/or treatment of obesity.

FRANK KONISHI

Carbondale, Illinois
25 April 1973

# Exercise Equivalents of Foods

# Suggested Weights for
# Varying Heights

13

One of the problems associated with the use of suggested
weight tables is the difficulty in defining the terms *ideal* or
*desirable*. For example, many individuals convince themselves
that their weights are "ideal" by interpreting weight tables ap-
propriately by claiming to have very large body frames. Unfortunately, a precise and simple method of estimating the size of
the body frame has not been established, so that it still remains
your prerogative to select your own body size. Actually, however,
the desirable weight may depend upon whether or not you are a
professional football player or a professional dancer. Since it has
not been possible to develop suitable tables which consider all
factors affecting ideal body weight, or to adequately define ideal
weight, it is necessary to rely on suggested weight tables based
on height, for men and women, as shown in tables 1 and 2.[2]
It is important to remember that for the majority of individuals,
your "ideal" weight is what you *should* have weighed at twenty-
two years of age.

# Recommended Calories Per Day

The calorie requirements of an individual are influenced by
many factors such as body size, age, sex, amount of exercise,
climate, pregnancy, and lactation.[3] The calorie requirements are
greater for large individuals, individuals who exercise, during
pregnancy and lactation periods, and when the temperature gets
cold (if not dressed properly) or extremely hot. On the other hand,

# 1. Suggested weights for men by height and body frame*

| Height In. (cm) | Small frame lbs. (kg) | | Average frame lbs. (kg) | | Large frame lbs. (kg) | |
|---|---|---|---|---|---|---|
| 60 (152) | 106 | (48) | 117 | (53) | 130 | (59) |
| 61 (155) | 110 | (50) | 121 | (55) | 133 | (60) |
| 62 (157) | 114 | (52) | 125 | (57) | 137 | (62) |
| 63 (160) | 118 | (54) | 129 | (59) | 141 | (64) |
| 64 (163) | 122 | (55) | 133 | (60) | 145 | (66) |
| 65 (165) | 126 | (57) | 137 | (62) | 149 | (68) |
| 66 (168) | 130 | (59) | 142 | (64) | 155 | (70) |
| 67 (170) | 134 | (61) | 147 | (67) | 161 | (73) |
| 68 (173) | 139 | (63) | 151 | (69) | 166 | (75) |
| 69 (175) | 143 | (65) | 155 | (70) | 170 | (77) |
| 70 (178) | 147 | (67) | 159 | (72) | 174 | (79) |
| 71 (180) | 150 | (68) | 163 | (74) | 178 | (81) |
| 72 (183) | 154 | (70) | 167 | (76) | 183 | (83) |
| 73 (185) | 158 | (72) | 171 | (78) | 188 | (85) |
| 74 (188) | 162 | (74) | 175 | (79) | 192 | (87) |
| 75 (191) | 165 | (75) | 178 | (81) | 195 | (89) |
| 76 (193) † | 168 | (76) | 181 | (82) | 198 | (90) |
| 77 (196) † | 172 | (78) | 185 | (84) | 202 | (92) |
| 78 (198) † | 175 | (80) | 188 | (86) | 205 | (93) |

*Without shoes and other clothing. Adapted from M. L. Hathaway and E. D. Foard, *Heights and Weights of Adults in the United States*, Home Economics Research Report No. 10 (Washington, D.C.: U.S. Department of Agriculture, 1960).
†Extrapolated values.

## 2. Suggested weights for women by height and body frame *

| Height In. (cm) | Small frame lbs. (kg) | | Average frame lbs. (kg) | | Large frame lbs. (kg) | |
|---|---|---|---|---|---|---|
| 58 (147) † | 94 | (43) | 102 | (46) | 110 | (50) |
| 59 (150) † | 97 | (44) | 105 | (48) | 114 | (52) |
| 60 (152) | 100 | (45) | 109 | (49) | 118 | (54) |
| 61 (155) | 104 | (47) | 112 | (51) | 121 | (55) |
| 62 (157) | 107 | (49) | 115 | (52) | 125 | (57) |
| 63 (160) | 110 | (50) | 118 | (54) | 128 | (58) |
| 64 (163) | 113 | (51) | 122 | (55) | 132 | (60) |
| 65 (165) | 116 | (53) | 125 | (57) | 135 | (61) |
| 66 (168) | 120 | (54) | 129 | (59) | 139 | (63) |
| 67 (170) | 123 | (56) | 132 | (60) | 142 | (64) |
| 68 (173) | 126 | (57) | 136 | (62) | 146 | (66) |
| 69 (175) | 130 | (59) | 140 | (64) | 151 | (69) |
| 70 (178) | 133 | (60) | 144 | (65) | 156 | (71) |
| 71 (180) | 137 | (62) | 148 | (67) | 161 | (73) |
| 72 (183) | 141 | (64) | 152 | (69) | 166 | (75) |
| 73 (185) | 145 | (66) | 156 | (71) | 171 | (78) |
| 74 (188) | 149 | (68) | 160 | (73) | 176 | (80) |
| 75 (191) | 153 | (69) | 164 | (74) | 181 | (82) |

*Without shoes and other clothing. Adapted from Hathaway and Foard.
†Extrapolated values.

---

the calorie requirements are smaller for women (because they may be smaller), for young and short people, and for sedentary people.

Tables 3 and 4 illustrate suggested calorie needs for adult men and women according to their body weights and ages. Notice that the requirements decrease with age. One reason many people become overweight as they grow older is because they continue to eat as much or the same at sixty-five years of age as they used to eat when they were twenty-two. This means that you should eat less as you grow older even if you can afford to buy more (remember, executive-type luncheons are usually high in calories). The ideal weight to try to maintain as you grow older is what you weighed (or should have weighed) at twenty-two years of age.

# Maintenance of Body Weight

Basically, when food or calorie intake equals calorie output or expenditure, body weight is maintained at a given level. However, if you have a tendency toward putting on weight, you should either decrease your calorie intake, exercise more, or do both. Maintenance of body weight by decreasing calorie intake is illustrated in table 5. The table shows the number of days it will take to lose 5 to 25 pounds when you decrease your calorie intake by 100 to 1,500 Cal each day below the level of calorie intake necessary to maintain your present weight, however overweight you may be. But if you are still gaining weight because you are eating 500 Cal each day in excess of those needed to maintain your present weight, deduct 500 Cal in addition to that recommended in table 5. This is a common error made by many individuals, who fail to consider how much they are really overeating.

## 3. Recommended calories per day for men by weight and age *

| Body weight | | Cal per day Age (in years) | | | | |
|---|---|---|---|---|---|---|
| lbs. | (kg) | 22 | 35 | 45 | 55 | 65 |
| 110 | (50) | 2,200 | 2,100 | 2,000 | 1,950 | 1,850 |
| 120 | (54) | 2,350 | 2,250 | 2,150 | 2,100 | 1,950 |
| 130 | (59) | 2,500 | 2,400 | 2,300 | 2,250 | 2,100 |
| 145 | (66) | 2,650 | 2,500 | 2,400 | 2,350 | 2,200 |
| 155 | (70) | 2,800 | 2,650 | 2,600 | 2,500 | 2,400 |
| 165 | (75) | 2,950 | 2,800 | 2,700 | 2,600 | 2,500 |
| 175 | (79) | 3,050 | 2,900 | 2,800 | 2,700 | 2,600 |
| 190 | (86) | 3,200 | 3,050 | 2,950 | 2,850 | 2,700 |
| 200 | (91) | 3,350 | 3,200 | 3,100 | 3,000 | 2,800 |
| 210 | (95) | 3,500 | 3,300 | 3,200 | 3,100 | 2,900 |
| 220 | (100) | 3,700 | 3,500 | 3,400 | 3,300 | 3,100 |
| 230 | (105) | 3,850 | 3,650 | 3,550 | 3,450 | 3,250 |
| 240 | (109) | 4,000 | 3,800 | 3,700 | 3,600 | 3,400 |
| 250 | (114) | 4,150 | 3,950 | 3,850 | 3,750 | 3,550 |

*Adapted from National Research Council, *Recommended Dietary Allowances*, 7th ed. (Washington, D.C.: National Academy of Sciences, 1968).

## 4. Recommended calories per day for women by weight and age *

| Body weight | | Cal per day | | | | |
| lbs. | (kg) | Age (in years) | | | | |
| | | 22 | 35 | 45 | 55 | 65 |
|---|---|---|---|---|---|---|
| 90 | (41) | 1,550 | 1,500 | 1,450 | 1,400 | 1,300 |
| 100 | (45) | 1,700 | 1,600 | 1,550 | 1,500 | 1,450 |
| 110 | (50) | 1,800 | 1,700 | 1,650 | 1,600 | 1,500 |
| 120 | (54) | 1,950 | 1,850 | 1,800 | 1,750 | 1,650 |
| 130 | (59) | 2,000 | 1,900 | 1,850 | 1,800 | 1,700 |
| 135 | (61) | 2,050 | 1,950 | 1,900 | 1,850 | 1,700 |
| 145 | (66) | 2,200 | 2,100 | 2,000 | 1,950 | 1,850 |
| 155 | (70) | 2,300 | 2,200 | 2,100 | 2,050 | 1,950 |
| 165 | (75) | 2,400 | 2,300 | 2,200 | 2,150 | 2,000 |
| 175 | (79) | 2,500 | 2,400 | 2,300 | 2,200 | 2,100 |
| 185 | (84) | 2,600 | 2,500 | 2,400 | 2,300 | 2,200 |
| 200 | (90) | 2,800 | 2,650 | 2,600 | 2,500 | 2,350 |

*Adapted from National Research Council, *Recommended Dietary Allowances*.

18

# 5. Days required to lose 5 to 25 pounds by lowering daily calorie intake

| Reduction of calories per day (in kcal) | Days to lose 5 lbs. | Days to lose 10 lbs. | Days to lose 15 lbs. | Days to lose 20 lbs. | Days to lose 25 lbs. |
|---|---|---|---|---|---|
| 100 | 150 | 300 | 450 | 600 | 750 |
| 200 | 75 | 150 | 225 | 300 | 375 |
| 300 | 50 | 100 | 150 | 200 | 250 |
| 400 | 38 | 75 | 114 | 150 | 190 |
| 500 | 30 | 60 | 90 | 120 | 150 |
| 600 | 25 | 50 | 75 | 100 | 125 |
| 700 | 22 | 44 | 66 | 88 | 110 |
| 800 | 19 | 38 | 57 | 75 | 95 |
| 900 | 17 | 34 | 51 | 68 | 85 |
| 1,000 | 15 | 30 | 45 | 60 | 75 |
| 1,200 | 11 | 22 | 33 | 44 | 55 |
| 1,500 | 5 | 10 | 15 | 20 | 25 |

20

The daily calorie intake must be lowered to that below the calorie intake recommended for maintenance of body weight (given in tables 3 and 4). The caloric value of body weight loss was calculated on the basis of 6,500 Cal/kg body fat or approximately 3,000 Cal/lb. of body fat. These are average values based on experiments reported by Keys and Grande.[4] It is known that the caloric equivalent of weight loss increases with the duration of the calorie restriction period. This is due to the fact that the body tends to lose more water than fat during the first few days of a reducing period. For example, the initial weight loss may have a caloric value of only 2,200 Cal/kg, while after 21 days the value may be as high as 8,700 Cal/kg.

# Exercise and Weight Loss

Ultimately, reductions in the rate of metabolism, overeating habits, and a decrease in amount of exercise are probably the major reasons why a person becomes overweight. As people get older the rate of metabolism decreases; they tend to exercise less; and they continue to eat as before; all of which favors a positive calorie balance and obesity. Proper exercise, then, is a good way of expending those extra calories and may permit you to continue to eat more of your favorite foods without putting on extra weight. Attempting to lose weight by exercise alone, however, is a very inefficient and discouraging process and is not recommended. A combination of a sensible exercise and calorie restriction program is recommended. Tables 6, 7, 8, 9, and 10 illustrate how different exercises for varying periods of time and a reduction in calories can assist you in losing 5 to 25 pounds. It should be emphasized that you not become discouraged when you see the number of days it takes to lose weight. It is well to

# 6. Days required to lose 5 to 25 pounds by walking * and lowering daily calorie intake

| Minutes of + walking | Reduction of calories per day (in kcal) | Days to lose 5 lbs. | Days to lose 10 lbs. | Days to lose 15 lbs. | Days to lose 20 lbs. | Days to lose 25 lbs. |
|---|---|---|---|---|---|---|
| 30 | 400 | 27 | 54 | 81 | 108 | 135 |
| 30 | 600 | 20 | 40 | 60 | 80 | 100 |
| 30 | 800 | 16 | 32 | 48 | 64 | 80 |
| 30 | 1,000 | 13 | 26 | 39 | 52 | 65 |
| 45 | 400 | 23 | 46 | 69 | 92 | 115 |
| 45 | 600 | 18 | 36 | 54 | 72 | 90 |
| 45 | 800 | 14 | 28 | 42 | 56 | 70 |
| 45 | 1,000 | 12 | 24 | 36 | 48 | 60 |
| 60 | 400 | 21 | 42 | 63 | 84 | 105 |
| 60 | 600 | 16 | 32 | 48 | 64 | 80 |
| 60 | 800 | 13 | 26 | 39 | 52 | 65 |
| 60 | 1,000 | 11 | 22 | 33 | 44 | 55 |

* Walking briskly (3.5–4.0 mph), calculated at 5.2 Cal/minute.

# 7. Days required to lose 5 to 25 pounds by bicycling * and lowering daily calorie intake

| Minutes of + bicycling | Reduction of calories per day (in kcal) | Days to lose 5 lbs. | Days to lose 10 lbs. | Days to lose 15 lbs. | Days to lose 20 lbs. | Days to lose 25 lbs. |
|---|---|---|---|---|---|---|
| 30 | 400 | 25 | 50 | 75 | 100 | 125 |
| 30 | 600 | 19 | 38 | 57 | 76 | 95 |
| 30 | 800 | 17 | 34 | 51 | 68 | 85 |
| 30 | 1,000 | 13 | 26 | 39 | 52 | 65 |
| 45 | 400 | 22 | 44 | 66 | 88 | 110 |
| 45 | 600 | 17 | 34 | 51 | 68 | 85 |
| 45 | 800 | 14 | 28 | 42 | 56 | 70 |
| 45 | 1,000 | 12 | 24 | 36 | 48 | 60 |
| 60 | 400 | 19 | 38 | 57 | 76 | 95 |
| 60 | 600 | 15 | 30 | 45 | 60 | 75 |
| 60 | 800 | 13 | 26 | 39 | 52 | 65 |
| 60 | 1,000 | 11 | 22 | 33 | 44 | 55 |

*Bicycling calculated at 6.5 Cal/minute, at approximately 7 mph.

# 8. Days required to lose 5 to 25 pounds by stepping * and lowering daily calorie intake

| Minutes of + stepping | Reduction of calories per day (in kcal) | Days to lose 5 lbs. | Days to lose 10 lbs. | Days to lose 15 lbs. | Days to lose 20 lbs. | Days to lose 25 lbs. |
|---|---|---|---|---|---|---|
| 30 | 400 | 24 | 48 | 72 | 96 | 120 |
| 30 | 600 | 18 | 36 | 54 | 72 | 90 |
| 30 | 800 | 15 | 30 | 45 | 60 | 75 |
| 30 | 1,000 | 12 | 24 | 36 | 48 | 60 |
| 45 | 400 | 20 | 40 | 60 | 80 | 100 |
| 45 | 600 | 16 | 32 | 48 | 64 | 80 |
| 45 | 800 | 13 | 26 | 39 | 52 | 65 |
| 45 | 1,000 | 11 | 22 | 33 | 44 | 55 |
| 60 | 400 | 18 | 36 | 54 | 72 | 90 |
| 60 | 600 | 14 | 28 | 42 | 56 | 70 |
| 60 | 800 | 12 | 24 | 36 | 48 | 60 |
| 60 | 1,000 | 10 | 20 | 30 | 40 | 50 |

* Stepping up and down on a regular 7″ step at 25 steps/minute, calculated at 7.5 Cal/minute.

## 9. Days required to lose 5 to 25 pounds by swimming * and lowering daily calorie intake

| Minutes of swimming | Reduction of calories per day (in kcal) | Days to lose 5 lbs | Days to lose 10 lbs. | Days to lose 15 lbs. | Days to lose 20 lbs. | Days to lose 25 lbs. |
|---|---|---|---|---|---|---|
| 30 | 400 | 23 | 46 | 69 | 92 | 115 |
| 30 | 600 | 18 | 36 | 52 | 72 | 90 |
| 30 | 800 | 14 | 28 | 42 | 56 | 70 |
| 30 | 1,000 | 12 | 24 | 36 | 48 | 60 |
| 45 | 400 | 19 | 38 | 57 | 76 | 95 |
| 45 | 600 | 15 | 30 | 45 | 60 | 75 |
| 45 | 800 | 13 | 26 | 39 | 52 | 65 |
| 45 | 1,000 | 11 | 22 | 33 | 44 | 55 |
| 60 | 400 | 16 | 32 | 48 | 64 | 80 |
| 60 | 600 | 14 | 28 | 42 | 56 | 70 |
| 60 | 800 | 11 | 22 | 33 | 44 | 55 |
| 60 | 1,000 | 10 | 20 | 30 | 40 | 50 |

*Swimming at about 30 yards/minute calculated at 8.5 Cal/minute.

## 10. Days required to lose 5 to 25 pounds by jogging * and lowering daily calorie intake

| Minutes of jogging | Reduction of calories per day (in kcal) | Days to lose 5 lbs. | Days to lose 10 lbs. | Days to lose 15 lbs. | Days to lose 20 lbs. | Days to lose 25 lbs. |
|---|---|---|---|---|---|---|
| 30 | 400 | 21 | 42 | 63 | 84 | 105 |
| 30 | 600 | 17 | 34 | 51 | 68 | 85 |
| 30 | 800 | 14 | 28 | 42 | 56 | 70 |
| 30 | 1,000 | 12 | 24 | 36 | 48 | 60 |
| 45 | 400 | 18 | 36 | 54 | 72 | 90 |
| 45 | 600 | 14 | 28 | 42 | 56 | 70 |
| 45 | 800 | 12 | 24 | 36 | 48 | 60 |
| 45 | 1,000 | 10 | 20 | 30 | 40 | 50 |
| 60 | 400 | 15 | 30 | 45 | 60 | 75 |
| 60 | 600 | 12 | 24 | 36 | 48 | 60 |
| 60 | 800 | 11 | 22 | 33 | 44 | 55 |
| 60 | 1,000 | 9 | 18 | 27 | 36 | 45 |

* Jogging—Alternate jogging and walking, calculated at 10.0 Cal/minute.

# Exercise and Weight Loss

remember that it probably took many more days to put on that extra weight, and it is unwise to try to lose it too quickly. The body requires time to adjust to the new pattern of eating and exercising.

Many forms of exercise can be recommended and the preferred type, of course, will vary from individual to individual. There are some basic factors to consider, however, in selecting a particular exercise. Such things as simplicity (not requiring special skills or equipment), sensitivity (being able to do them in the privacy of one's home or immediate vicinity), and sensibility (not too strenuous and with the advice of your physician) are important aspects to take into consideration. The exercises selected for purposes of this book fulfil these requirements and can be adopted singly or in combination for a body weight-control program. The exercises are presented in increasing order of energy cost or work.

It is realized that the energy costs of the various activities will vary considerably among individuals and therefore should not be viewed as an absolute value. The energy costs of all the activities, except swimming, will be higher for the heavier individual. Unfortunately, many values in the available literature are based on the reference man, i.e., 154 lbs. or 70 kg in weight and 5'9" or 175 cm tall. If you weigh more than the reference man, your caloric costs may be higher and if you weigh less, your caloric costs may be lower. It is recognized, therefore, that the energy cost values in this book are average values and should be used accordingly. Finally, in any weight reduction program where calorie restriction is recommended, it is imperative that the intakes of the essential vitamins, minerals, protein, and water be maintained at the levels recommended by the National Research Council[5] and your physician.

---

# Walking

Walking briskly at 3.5 to 4.0 mph at an average cost of 5.2 Cal/minute.[6] This rate of caloric expenditure approximates the level at which the majority of individuals should be able to perform for up to eight hours without incurring an oxygen debt. Very few people, however, would have the time or inclination to walk for eight hours! The calorie cost will vary according to your weight, type of shoe, type of surface, and the terrain.

# Bicycling

This is an enjoyable form of exercise that can consume around 6.5 Cal/minute (at about 7 mph) as well as to provide an opportunity to see a lot of country (or city) for people of all ages.[7] The calorie cost, of course, will vary depending upon the terrain, type of surface, type of bicycle, speed, efficiency, skill, and so forth.

# Stepping

This activity can be performed anywhere where there is a standard seven-inch step or stool available. The procedure is to step up onto the step and then step down. The suggested rate is 25 up and down steps/minute while facing the same direction. The amount of work required for stepping will average about 7.5 Cal/minute.

## Swimming

The energy cost of swimming will vary considerably depending upon your skill while in the water. If you are an average swimmer (30 yards/minute), however, this is an excellent method of keeping in good physical condition while consuming approximately 8.5 Cal/minute.[8] If you are a poor swimmer, the caloric cost may be considerable higher.

## Jogging

The term is relatively recent but the activity has been around for years, as trotting. Since jogging may be too strenuous for some, especially the novice, it is recommended that the jogging be alternated with walking, for example, 5 minutes jogging + 5 minutes walking + 5 minutes jogging, and so forth. With this procedure, you will expend around 10.0 Cal/minute. The only special equipment required will be a comfortable pair of shoes.

## Exercise Equivalents of Food Calories

If you have ever wondered how long to exercise, what type of exercise to do, or whether or not you should eat that last remaining piece of cake, the exercise equivalents of foods listed in table 11 may help you decide. The table illustrates the number of

# Exercise Equivalents of Food Calories in Minutes

minutes to exercise (and which exercise to do) to expend an equivalent number of calories contained in a given food. The values in the table are designed to discourage the eating of excess food by relating the caloric content of a food in exercise units.

# 11. Exercise Equivalents of Food Calories in Minutes

**Table 11**

| FOOD | WEIGHT 1oz.=30gm | CALORIES | WALKING | BICYCLING | STEPPING | SWIMMING | JOGGING |
|---|---|---|---|---|---|---|---|
| | gm. | kcal. | min. | min. | min. | min. | min. |
| ALCOHOLIC BEVERAGES | | | | | | | |
| Ale<br>8 oz. glass | 230 | 100 | 19 | 15 | 13 | 12 | 10 |
| Apricot brandy<br>1 cordial glass | 20 | 65 | 12 | 10 | 9 | 8 | 7 |
| Beer<br>8 oz. glass | 240 | 115 | 22 | 18 | 15 | 14 | 12 |
| Benedictine<br>1 cordial glass | 20 | 70 | 13 | 11 | 9 | 8 | 7 |
| Brandy-California<br>1 brandy glass | 30 | 75 | 14 | 12 | 10 | 9 | 8 |
| Brandy-cognac<br>1 brandy pony | 30 | 75 | 14 | 12 | 10 | 9 | 8 |
| Cider, fermented<br>6 oz. glass | 180 | 70 | 13 | 10 | 9 | 8 | 7 |
| Cordial-Anisette<br>1 cordial glass | 20 | 75 | 14 | 12 | 10 | 9 | 8 |
| Creme de menthe<br>1 cordial glass | 20 | 68 | 13 | 10 | 9 | 8 | 7 |
| Curacao<br>1 cordial glass | 20 | 68 | 13 | 10 | 9 | 8 | 7 |
| Daiquiri<br>1 cocktail glass | 100 | 125 | 24 | 19 | 17 | 15 | 13 |
| Eggnog<br>4 oz. punch cup | 120 | 335 | 64 | 53 | 45 | 39 | 34 |

*One ounce has been rounded to equal 30 grams.

†Values based on data from C. F. Church and H. N. Church, *Food Values of Portions Commonly Used*, 11th ed. (Philadelphia: J. B. Lippincott, 1970); B. K. Watt and A. L. Merrill, *Composition of Foods,* USDA Handbook No. 8 (Washington, D.C., 1963); USDA *Nutritive Value of Foods,* Home and Garden Bulletin No. 72, USDA, ARS (Washington, D.C., 1971). Calories listed are in kilocalories.

# Table 11 (cont.)

| FOOD | WEIGHT 1oz.=30gm gm. | CALORIES kcal. | WALKING min. | BICYCLING min. | STEPPING min. | SWIMMING min. | JOGGING min. |
|---|---|---|---|---|---|---|---|
| Gin, dry<br>1½ oz., 1 jigger | 43 | 105 | 20 | 16 | 14 | 12 | 11 |
| Gin rickey<br>1 glass | 120 | 150 | 29 | 23 | 20 | 18 | 15 |
| High ball<br>8 oz. glass | 240 | 165 | 32 | 25 | 22 | 19 | 17 |
| Manhattan, cocktail<br>3½ oz. | 100 | 165 | 32 | 25 | 22 | 19 | 17 |
| Martini, cocktail<br>3½ oz. | 100 | 140 | 27 | 22 | 19 | 16 | 14 |
| Mint julep<br>10 oz. glass | 300 | 215 | 41 | 33 | 29 | 25 | 22 |
| Muscatelle, port<br>3½ oz. glass | 100 | 160 | 31 | 25 | 21 | 19 | 16 |
| Old fashioned<br>4 oz. glass | 120 | 180 | 35 | 28 | 24 | 21 | 18 |
| Planter's punch<br>1 glass | 100 | 175 | 34 | 27 | 23 | 21 | 18 |
| Rum<br>1 jigger, 1½ oz. | 45 | 105 | 20 | 16 | 14 | 12 | 11 |
| Sauterne, California<br>3½ oz. glass | 100 | 85 | 16 | 13 | 11 | 10 | 9 |
| Scotch<br>1 jigger, 1½ oz. | 45 | 105 | 20 | 16 | 14 | 12 | 11 |
| Sherry<br>2 oz. glass | 60 | 85 | 16 | 13 | 11 | 10 | 9 |
| Tom Collins<br>10 oz. glass | 300 | 180 | 35 | 28 | 24 | 21 | 18 |
| Vermouth, French<br>3½ oz. glass | 100 | 105 | 20 | 16 | 14 | 12 | 11 |

# Exercise Equivalents of Food Calories in Minutes

## Table 11 (cont.)

| FOOD | WEIGHT 1oz.=30gm gm. | CALORIES kcal. | WALKING min. | BICYCLING min. | STEPPING min. | SWIMMING min. | JOGGING min. |
|---|---|---|---|---|---|---|---|
| Vermouth, Italian 3½ oz. glass | 100 | 170 | 33 | 26 | 23 | 20 | 17 |
| Whiskey, Bourbon, rye 1 jigger, 1½ oz. | 45 | 120 | 23 | 18 | 16 | 14 | 12 |
| Wine, Burgundy 4 oz. glass | 120 | 110 | 21 | 16 | 15 | 13 | 11 |
| Wine, Champagne 4 oz. glass | 120 | 85 | 16 | 13 | 11 | 10 | 9 |
| Wine, Port 4 oz. glass | 120 | 210 | 40 | 32 | 28 | 25 | 21 |
| | | | | | | | |
| BEVERAGES | | | | | | | |
| Carbonated, average 6 oz. bottle | 180 | 80 | 15 | 12 | 11 | 9 | 8 |
| Coca-Cola 8 oz. glass | 240 | 105 | 20 | 16 | 14 | 12 | 11 |
| Gingerale 8 oz. glass | 240 | 80 | 14 | 12 | 11 | 9 | 8 |
| Pepsi-Cola 8 oz. glass | 240 | 105 | 20 | 16 | 14 | 12 | 11 |
| Chocolate milk 1 teacup (6½ oz.) | 200 | 210 | 40 | 32 | 28 | 25 | 21 |
| Cider, sweet 8 oz. glass | 240 | 124 | 24 | 19 | 17 | 15 | 12 |
| Cocoa, all milk 1 teacup (6½ oz.) | 200 | 175 | 34 | 27 | 23 | 21 | 18 |
| Coffee & sugar 1 cup; 1 tsp. | 200 | 30 | 6 | 5 | 4 | 4 | 3 |
| Coffee, Sugar & Cream 1 cup; 1 tsp. & 1 tbs. | 220 | 62 | 12 | 10 | 8 | 7 | 6 |

# Table 11 (cont.)

| FOOD | WEIGHT 1oz.=30gm gm. | CALORIES kcal. | WALKING min. | BICYCLING min. | STEPPING min. | SWIMMING min. | JOGGING min. |
|---|---|---|---|---|---|---|---|
| Eggnog<br>6 oz. glass | 240 | 235 | 45 | 36 | 31 | 28 | 24 |
| Lemonade<br>1 glass | 290 | 105 | 20 | 16 | 14 | 12 | 11 |
| Milk, chocolate<br>8 oz. glass | 240 | 205 | 39 | 32 | 27 | 24 | 21 |
| Milk, malted<br>12 oz. glass | 365 | 500 | 96 | 77 | 67 | 59 | 50 |
| Milk, whole<br>8 oz. glass | 240 | 160 | 31 | 25 | 21 | 19 | 16 |
| Milk shake<br>12 oz. glass | 345 | 420 | 81 | 65 | 56 | 49 | 42 |
| Ovaltine<br>8 oz. glass | 260 | 220 | 42 | 34 | 29 | 26 | 22 |
| Postum, instant<br>1 cup | 185 | 36 | 7 | 6 | 5 | 4 | 4 |
| Soda, ice cream (vanilla)<br>1 regular (8 oz.) | 240 | 255 | 49 | 39 | 34 | 30 | 26 |
| Tea & sugar<br>1 cup; 1 tsp. | 200 | 25 | 5 | 4 | 3 | 3 | 3 |
| Tea, sugar & cream<br>1 cup; 1 tsp.; 1 tbs. | 220 | 57 | 11 | 9 | 8 | 7 | 6 |
| **BREADS** | | | | | | | |
| Bread (fresh or toasted;<br>(White, rye, whole wheat,<br>Italian, French)<br>1 slice | 23 | 60 | 12 | 9 | 8 | 7 | 6 |
| Bread, banana<br>1 slice ($3\frac{1}{2}'' \times 3\frac{1}{2}'' \times \frac{3}{8}''$) | 50 | 135 | 26 | 21 | 18 | 16 | 14 |

# Exercise Equivalents of Food Calories in Minutes

## Table 11 (cont.)

| FOOD | WEIGHT 1oz.=30gm gm. | CALORIES kcal. | WALKING min. | BICYCLING min. | STEPPING min. | SWIMMING min. | JOGGING min. |
|---|---|---|---|---|---|---|---|
| Bread, banana with butter<br>1 slice; 1 pat * | 55 | 170 | 33 | 26 | 23 | 20 | 17 |
| Bread, buttered<br>1 slice; 1 pat | 28 | 96 | 18 | 15 | 13 | 11 | 10 |
| Bread, butter & jam<br>1 slice; 1 pat; 1 tsp. | 33 | 106 | 20 | 16 | 14 | 12 | 11 |
| Bread, nut<br>1 slice | 50 | 135 | 26 | 21 | 18 | 16 | 14 |
| Bread, peanut butter<br>1 slice; 1/2 tbs. | 33 | 102 | 20 | 16 | 14 | 12 | 10 |
| Bread, peanut butter & jam<br>1 slice; 1/2 tbs.; 1 tsp. | 38 | 112 | 22 | 17 | 15 | 13 | 11 |
| Biscuit<br>2″ diam. | 35 | 130 | 25 | 20 | 17 | 15 | 13 |
| Biscuit, buttered<br>2″ diam.; 1 pat | 40 | 166 | 32 | 26 | 22 | 20 | 17 |
| Biscuit, buttered with honey<br>2″ diam.; 1 pat; 1 tsp. | 45 | 200 | 38 | 31 | 27 | 24 | 20 |
| Biscuit, honey<br>2″ diam.; 1 tsp. | 40 | 164 | 32 | 25 | 22 | 19 | 16 |
| Biscuit, jam<br>2″ diam.; 1 tsp. | 40 | 140 | 27 | 22 | 19 | 16 | 14 |
| Muffin<br>1 plain | 40 | 120 | 23 | 18 | 16 | 14 | 12 |
| Muffin, buttered<br>1 plain | 45 | 154 | 30 | 24 | 21 | 18 | 15 |
| Muffin, blueberry<br>1 plain | 40 | 112 | 22 | 17 | 15 | 13 | 11 |
| Muffin, english, buttered<br>4″ diam.; 1 pat | 60 | 180 | 34 | 28 | 24 | 22 | 18 |

* 1 pat = 5 grams = 1 tsp.

**Table 11 (cont.)**

| FOOD | WEIGHT 1oz.=30gm | CALORIES | WALKING | BICYCLING | STEPPING | SWIMMING | JOGGING |
|------|------|------|------|------|------|------|------|
| | gm. | kcal. | min. | min. | min. | min. | min. |
| Pancake<br>4″ diam. | 45 | 105 | 20 | 16 | 14 | 12 | 11 |
| Pancake, with butter & syrup<br>1 pat; 2 tbs. | 90 | 240 | 46 | 36 | 32 | 28 | 24 |
| Pancake & syrup<br>4″ diam.; 2 tbs. | 85 | 204 | 39 | 31 | 27 | 24 | 20 |
| Roll, hard<br>1 ave. | 35 | 109 | 21 | 16 | 15 | 13 | 11 |
| Roll, hard with butter<br>1 ave.; 1 pat | 40 | 145 | 28 | 22 | 19 | 17 | 15 |
| Roll, sweet<br>1 ave. | 55 | 180 | 35 | 27 | 24 | 21 | 18 |
| Toast, French with syrup<br>1 slice; 2 tbs. | 105 | 165 | 31 | 25 | 22 | 20 | 17 |
| Tortilla<br>6″ diam. | 30 | 65 | 13 | 10 | 9 | 8 | 7 |
| Waffle, plain<br>5½″ diam. | 75 | 210 | 40 | 32 | 28 | 25 | 21 |
| Waffle, butter & syrup<br>5½″ diam.; 1 pat; 2 tbsp. | 120 | 345 | 66 | 52 | 46 | 41 | 35 |
| **CANDY** | | | | | | | |
| Almond bar, chocolate<br>1 bar, 1¼ oz. | 38 | 310 | 60 | 46 | 41 | 36 | 31 |
| Butterscotch<br>5 pieces (90 pieces/lb.) | 25 | 100 | 19 | 15 | 13 | 12 | 10 |
| Candy, hard (all flavors)<br>1 oz. | 30 | 110 | 21 | 17 | 15 | 13 | 11 |
| Caramel<br>1 oz. | 30 | 118 | 23 | 18 | 16 | 14 | 12 |

# Exercise Equivalents of Food Calories in Minutes

**Table 11 (cont.)**

| FOOD | WEIGHT 1oz.=30gm | CALORIES | WALKING | BICYCLING | STEPPING | SWIMMING | JOGGING |
|------|------------------|----------|---------|-----------|----------|----------|---------|
| | gm. | kcal. | min. | min. | min. | min. | min. |
| Chocolate cream<br>1 piece (35/lb.) | 13 | 50 | 10 | 8 | 7 | 6 | 5 |
| Chocolate fudge<br>1¼″ square | 30 | 118 | 23 | 18 | 16 | 14 | 12 |
| Chocolate mint<br>1 small (45/lb.) | 10 | 40 | 8 | 6 | 5 | 5 | 4 |
| Forever Yours<br>1¾ oz. | 52 | 192 | 37 | 29 | 26 | 23 | 19 |
| Gum drops<br>8 small | 10 | 33 | 6 | 5 | 4 | 4 | 3 |
| Hershey bar<br>1⅜ oz. | 40 | 209 | 40 | 31 | 27 | 25 | 21 |
| Hershey chocolate kisses<br>7 pieces | 28 | 152 | 29 | 23 | 20 | 18 | 15 |
| Jelly beans<br>10 beans | 28 | 66 | 13 | 10 | 9 | 8 | 7 |
| Lollypops<br>1 med. | 28 | 108 | 21 | 16 | 14 | 13 | 11 |
| Mars bar<br>1⅜ oz. | 40 | 212 | 40 | 32 | 28 | 25 | 21 |
| Marshmallow<br>1 ave. (60/lb.) | 8 | 25 | 5 | 4 | 3 | 3 | 3 |
| Milky Way<br>1¾ oz. | 52 | 192 | 37 | 29 | 26 | 23 | 19 |
| Mints, cream<br>10 mints | 15 | 53 | 10 | 8 | 7 | 6 | 5 |
| Mr. Goodbar<br>1⅝ oz. | 48 | 250 | 48 | 38 | 32 | 29 | 25 |
| Peanut brittle<br>2½ × 2½ × ⅜″ | 25 | 110 | 21 | 16 | 15 | 13 | 11 |
| Peanut butter, chocolate covered<br>1 oz. | 30 | 135 | 26 | 21 | 18 | 15 | 14 |

**Table 11 (cont.)**

| FOOD | WEIGHT 1oz.=30gm | CALORIES | WALKING | BICYCLING | STEPPING | SWIMMING | JOGGING |
|---|---|---|---|---|---|---|---|
| | gm. | kcal. | min. | min. | min. | min. | min. |
| Snickers 1⅝ oz. | 48 | 174 | 33 | 26 | 23 | 20 | 17 |
| Three Musketeers 1¹⁵⁄₁₆ oz. | 58 | 207 | 39 | 31 | 27 | 24 | 21 |
| **CEREALS — BREAKFAST** | | | | | | | |
| Bran flakes, milk & sugar * ¾ cup; ½ cup; 1 tsp. | 153 | 212 | 41 | 32 | 28 | 25 | 21 |
| Bran, raisin, milk & sugar ⅔ cup; ½ cup; 1 tsp. | 153 | 212 | 41 | 32 | 28 | 25 | 21 |
| Cream of wheat, milk & sugar 1 cup; ½ cup; 1 tsp. | 163 | 245 | 47 | 37 | 33 | 29 | 25 |
| Oatmeal, milk & sugar 1 cup cooked; ¼ cup; 1 tsp. | 301 | 260 | 50 | 39 | 35 | 31 | 26 |
| Other cereals, ready to serve or hot, milk & sugar 1 cup; ½ cup; 1 tsp. | 153 | 212 | 41 | 32 | 28 | 25 | 21 |
| **CEREAL PRODUCTS** | | | | | | | |
| Macaroni, or pasta, cooked 1 cup | 140 | 205 | 39 | 31 | 27 | 24 | 21 |
| Macaroni & cheese 1 cup | 225 | 505 | 97 | 76 | 67 | 59 | 51 |
| Noodles, egg, cooked 1 cup | 160 | 200 | 38 | 30 | 27 | 24 | 20 |

\* ½ cup whole milk    1 tsp. sugar = 112 Calories
½ cup 2% milk    1 tsp. sugar = 95 Calories
½ cup skim milk    1 tsp. sugar = 76 Calories
Sugar would not be added to presweetened cereals.

# Exercise Equivalents of Food Calories in Minutes

## Table 11 (cont.)

| FOOD | WEIGHT 1oz.=30gm gm. | CALORIES kcal. | WALKING min. | BICYCLING min. | STEPPING min. | SWIMMING min. | JOGGING min. |
|---|---|---|---|---|---|---|---|
| Popcorn, butter & salt 1 cup; 1 tsp. | 18 | 82 | 16 | 12 | 11 | 10 | 8 |
| Popcorn, plain 1 cup | 14 | 54 | 10 | 8 | 7 | 6 | 5 |
| Rice, brown, cooked 1 cup | 150 | 178 | 34 | 27 | 24 | 21 | 18 |
| Rice, white, cooked 1 cup | 150 | 164 | 32 | 25 | 22 | 19 | 16 |
| Spaghetti, meat balls 1 serving | 220 | 295 | 57 | 44 | 39 | 35 | 30 |
| Spaghetti, meat sauce, Italian 1 serving | 292 | 396 | 76 | 59 | 53 | 47 | 40 |
| Spaghetti, tomato sauce 1 serving | 220 | 180 | 35 | 27 | 24 | 21 | 18 |
| Spanish rice, cooked 1 cup | 150 | 130 | 25 | 20 | 17 | 15 | 13 |
| COOKIES | | | | | | | |
| Chocolate chip 1 cookie (43/lb) | 11 | 50 | 10 | 8 | 7 | 6 | 5 |
| Chocolate snaps 5 (120/lb.) | 19 | 90 | 17 | 14 | 12 | 11 | 9 |
| Coconut bar 1 bar (32/lb) | 14 | 70 | 14 | 10 | 9 | 8 | 7 |
| Fig Newton 1 (31/lb.) | 15 | 55 | 11 | 8 | 7 | 6 | 6 |
| Ginger snaps 1 cookie | 11 | 30 | 6 | 5 | 4 | 4 | 3 |
| Golden sugar 1 (21/lb.) | 22 | 98 | 19 | 15 | 13 | 12 | 10 |

# Table 11 (cont.)

| FOOD | WEIGHT 1oz.=30gm gm. | CALORIES kcal. | WALKING min. | BICYCLING min. | STEPPING min. | SWIMMING min. | JOGGING min. |
|---|---|---|---|---|---|---|---|
| Nabisco sugar wafers 4 wafers | 12 | 60 | 11 | 9 | 8 | 7 | 6 |
| Oatmeal 1 (24/lb.) | 19 | 86 | 17 | 13 | 11 | 10 | 9 |
| Oreo creme 1 sandwich (39/lb.) | 12 | 40 | 8 | 6 | 5 | 5 | 4 |
| Peanut butter 1 cookie | 12 | 30 | 6 | 5 | 4 | 4 | 3 |
| Vanilla wafers 4 (142/lb.) | 13 | 60 | 11 | 9 | 8 | 7 | 6 |
| CRACKERS | | | | | | | |
| Animal (Barnum's) 10 crackers (225/lb.) | 20 | 90 | 17 | 14 | 12 | 11 | 9 |
| Blue cheese 5 crackers (212/lb.) | 10 | 55 | 11 | 8 | 7 | 6 | 6 |
| Cheese tidbits 10 crackers (1300/lb.) | 4 | 20 | 4 | 3 | 3 | 2 | 2 |
| Graham, Nabisco 1 cracker (65/lb) | 7 | 30 | 6 | 4 | 4 | 4 | 3 |
| Melba toast, unsalted 1 slice, thin | 4 | 15 | 3 | 2 | 2 | 2 | 2 |
| Oyster crackers 10 crackers | 7 | 30 | 6 | 5 | 4 | 4 | 3 |
| Pretzels, 3-ring 4 (148/lb.) | 12 | 48 | 9 | 7 | 6 | 6 | 5 |
| Pretzels, Veri-Thin sticks 10 sticks (1600/lb.) | 3 | 10 | 2 | 1 | 1 | 1 | 1 |
| Peanut butter cheese 1 (4/pack) | 8 | 39 | 8 | 6 | 5 | 5 | 4 |

# Exercise Equivalents of Food Calories in Minutes

**Table 11 (cont.)**

| FOOD | WEIGHT 1oz.=30gm | CALORIES | WALKING | BICYCLING | STEPPING | SWIMMING | JOGGING |
|------|------------------|----------|---------|-----------|----------|----------|---------|
|      | gm. | kcal. | min. | min. | min. | min. | min. |
| Ritz<br>4 crackers (138/lb.) | 13 | 68 | 13 | 10 | 9 | 8 | 7 |
| Ry-Krisp<br>2 crackers (36/lb.) | 13 | 42 | 8 | 6 | 6 | 5 | 4 |
| Rye thins<br>4 crackers (181/lb.) | 12 | 52 | 10 | 8 | 7 | 6 | 5 |
| Saltines<br>2 crackers (140/lb.) | 6 | 28 | 5 | 4 | 4 | 3 | 3 |
| Zwieback<br>2 pieces (62/lb.) | 15 | 62 | 12 | 9 | 8 | 7 | 6 |
| DAIRY PRODUCTS | | | | | | | |
| Butter<br>1 pat (1″ × 1″ × 1/3″) | 5 | 35 | 7 | 5 | 5 | 4 | 4 |
| Cheese, blue mold<br>1 oz. | 30 | 103 | 20 | 15 | 14 | 12 | 10 |
| Cheese, American<br>1 slice (1 oz.) | 30 | 112 | 22 | 17 | 15 | 13 | 11 |
| Cheese, Parmesan<br>1 oz. | 30 | 130 | 25 | 20 | 17 | 16 | 13 |
| Cheese spread<br>1 oz. | 30 | 80 | 15 | 12 | 11 | 9 | 8 |
| Cottage cheese<br>1 round tbs. | 30 | 30 | 6 | 4 | 4 | 4 | 3 |
| Cream<br>1 tbs. | 15 | 32 | 6 | 5 | 4 | 4 | 3 |
| Cream, sour, cultured<br>1 oz. | 30 | 57 | 11 | 9 | 8 | 7 | 6 |
| Cream, whipped<br>1 rd. tbs.; 1/2 tsp. sugar | 17 | 56 | 11 | 8 | 7 | 7 | 6 |

# Table 11 (cont.)

| FOOD | WEIGHT 1oz.=30gm gm. | CALORIES kcal. | WALKING min. | BICYCLING min. | STEPPING min. | SWIMMING min. | JOGGING min. |
|---|---|---|---|---|---|---|---|
| Ice cream<br>⅙ qt.; 5 rd. tbs. | 90 | 186 | 36 | 28 | 25 | 22 | 19 |
| Ice cream bar, choc. coated<br>1 bar | 60 | 195 | 37 | 30 | 26 | 23 | 20 |
| Ice cream bar, sherbet coated<br>1 bar | 60 | 96 | 18 | 15 | 13 | 12 | 10 |
| Ice cream cone<br>1 dip | 72 | 160 | 31 | 24 | 21 | 19 | 16 |
| Ice cream sandwich | 75 | 208 | 40 | 32 | 28 | 25 | 21 |
| Ice cream sundae<br>2 dips | 75 | 326 | 63 | 49 | 43 | 39 | 33 |
| Ice milk<br>⅙ qt.; 5 round tbs. | 90 | 137 | 26 | 21 | 18 | 16 | 14 |
| Ice milk bar choc. coated<br>1 bar | 60 | 144 | 27 | 22 | 19 | 17 | 14 |
| Milk, buttermilk<br>8 oz. glass | 240 | 88 | 17 | 13 | 12 | 10 | 9 |
| Milk, chocolate<br>8 oz. glass | 240 | 205 | 39 | 32 | 27 | 25 | 21 |
| Milk, skim<br>8 oz. glass | 240 | 88 | 17 | 13 | 12 | 10 | 9 |
| Milk, 2% fat<br>8 oz. glass | 240 | 126 | 24 | 19 | 17 | 15 | 13 |
| Milk, whole<br>8 oz. glass | 240 | 160 | 31 | 25 | 21 | 19 | 16 |
| Oleomargarine<br>1 tsp. | 5 | 36 | 7 | 5 | 5 | 4 | 4 |
| Yogurt, from skim milk<br>1 cup | 240 | 122 | 24 | 18 | 16 | 14 | 12 |

# Exercise Equivalents of Food Calories in Minutes

## Table 11 (cont.)

| FOOD | WEIGHT 1oz.=30gm | CALORIES | WALKING | BICYCLING | STEPPING | SWIMMING | JOGGING |
|---|---|---|---|---|---|---|---|
| | gm. | kcal. | min. | min. | min. | min. | min. |
| DESSERTS | | | | | | | |
| Banana split | 300 | 594 | 114 | 89 | 79 | 71 | 59 |
| Boston cream pie 1 serving | 110 | 332 | 64 | 50 | 44 | 39 | 33 |
| Brownies, with nuts 1 piece (2″ × 2″ × ¾″) | 30 | 146 | 28 | 22 | 19 | 17 | 15 |
| Cakes: | | | | | | | |
| Angel food 1 piece, 1/12 of 10″ cake | 53 | 135 | 26 | 20 | 18 | 16 | 14 |
| Caramel with icing 1 piece, 1/12 of 9″ cake | 55 | 208 | 40 | 31 | 28 | 24 | 21 |
| Chocolate with icing 1 piece (2″ × 3″ × 2″) | 55 | 205 | 39 | 31 | 27 | 24 | 21 |
| Cupcake with icing 1 (2½″ diam.) | 36 | 130 | 25 | 20 | 17 | 16 | 13 |
| Fruitcake 1 slice (3″ × 3″ × ½″) | 40 | 152 | 29 | 23 | 20 | 18 | 15 |
| Plain cake with icing 1 piece, 1/2 of 9″ cake | 50 | 186 | 36 | 28 | 25 | 22 | 19 |
| Pound cake 1 slice (3″ × 3″ × ½″) | 30 | 142 | 27 | 21 | 19 | 17 | 14 |
| White cake 1 piece, 1/12 of 9″ cake | 50 | 186 | 35 | 28 | 24 | 22 | 19 |
| Cake, with ice cream 1/12 of 9″; 1 dip | 110 | 301 | 57 | 45 | 39 | 36 | 30 |
| Cheesecake 1 slice, 1/12 of 9″ cake | 50 | 160 | 30 | 25 | 21 | 19 | 16 |
| Custard, baked 1 custard | 157 | 205 | 39 | 31 | 27 | 24 | 21 |
| Doughnut 1 average | 32 | 125 | 24 | 19 | 17 | 15 | 13 |

# Table 11 (cont.)

| FOOD | WEIGHT 1oz.=30gm gm. | CALORIES kcal. | WALKING min. | BICYCLING min. | STEPPING min. | SWIMMING min. | JOGGING min. |
|------|------|------|------|------|------|------|------|
| Doughnut, jelly center 1 average | 65 | 226 | 44 | 34 | 30 | 27 | 23 |
| Eclair or cream puff 1 average | 105 | 296 | 57 | 44 | 39 | 35 | 30 |
| Ice cream 1 dip | 60 | 115 | 22 | 17 | 15 | 14 | 12 |
| Jello, plain 1 serving (5/pkg) | 65 | 65 | 13 | 10 | 9 | 8 | 7 |
| Jello, with whipped cream 1 serving; 1 tbs. | 80 | 117 | 23 | 18 | 16 | 14 | 12 |
| Parfait, coffee 1 serving | 107 | 258 | 50 | 39 | 34 | 30 | 26 |
| Pies (⅙ of 9″ pie): | | | | | | | |
|   Banana custard | 160 | 355 | 68 | 53 | 47 | 42 | 36 |
|   Butterscotch | 160 | 430 | 83 | 64 | 57 | 51 | 43 |
|   Chocolate chiffon | 160 | 525 | 101 | 79 | 70 | 62 | 53 |
|   Chocolate meringue | 150 | 380 | 73 | 57 | 50 | 45 | 38 |
|   Coconut custard | 155 | 365 | 70 | 55 | 48 | 43 | 37 |
|   Fruit pies | 160 | 400 | 77 | 60 | 53 | 47 | 40 |
|   Fruit pies, ala mode | 220 | 515 | 99 | 77 | 68 | 62 | 52 |
|   Pecan | 160 | 670 | 129 | 100 | 89 | 78 | 67 |
|   Lemon chiffon | 107 | 335 | 64 | 50 | 45 | 39 | 34 |
|   Pumpkin | 150 | 320 | 62 | 48 | 42 | 38 | 32 |
| Popsicle | 95 | 70 | 14 | 10 | 9 | 8 | 7 |
| Pudding, bread with raisins ¾ cup | 165 | 315 | 61 | 47 | 42 | 37 | 32 |
| Pudding, chocolate ½ cup | 130 | 192 | 36 | 29 | 25 | 23 | 19 |
| Rice pudding with raisins ¾ cup | 145 | 212 | 41 | 32 | 28 | 25 | 21 |

# Exercise Equivalents of Food Calories in Minutes

**Table 11 (cont.)**

| FOOD | WEIGHT 1oz.=30gm | CALORIES | WALKING | BICYCLING | STEPPING | SWIMMING | JOGGING |
|---|---|---|---|---|---|---|---|
| | gm. | kcal. | min. | min. | min. | min. | min. |
| Sherbet, orange<br>1/6 qt., 5 tbs. | 90 | 120 | 23 | 18 | 16 | 14 | 12 |
| Shortcake, peach slices<br>1 biscuit, 1 peach | 150 | 266 | 51 | 40 | 35 | 31 | 27 |
| **EGGS** | | | | | | | |
| Boiled or poached<br>1 med. | 48 | 78 | 15 | 12 | 10 | 9 | 8 |
| Fried or scrambled<br>1 med.; 1 tsp. oil | 53 | 108 | 21 | 16 | 14 | 13 | 11 |
| Omelet, plain egg<br>1 med.; 1 tsp. oil | 53 | 107 | 21 | 16 | 14 | 13 | 11 |
| White only | 31 | 18 | 3 | 3 | 2 | 2 | 2 |
| Yolk only | 17 | 60 | 11 | 9 | 8 | 7 | 6 |
| **FRUITS** | | | | | | | |
| Apple, raw<br>1 med. (2½" diam) | 150 | 87 | 17 | 13 | 12 | 10 | 9 |
| Apple, baked<br>1 med.; 2 tbs. sugar | 150 | 188 | 36 | 28 | 25 | 22 | 19 |
| Applesauce<br>1/3 cup | 100 | 90 | 17 | 14 | 12 | 11 | 9 |
| Apricots, canned (water pack)<br>3 havles | 100 | 38 | 7 | 6 | 5 | 4 | 4 |
| Apricots, raw<br>3 med. | 100 | 50 | 10 | 8 | 7 | 6 | 5 |

# Table 11 (cont.)

| FOOD | WEIGHT 1oz.=30gm | CALORIES | WALKING | BICYCLING | STEPPING | SWIMMING | JOGGING |
|---|---|---|---|---|---|---|---|
| | gm. | kcal. | min. | min. | min. | min. | min. |
| Avocado, raw<br>1/2 pitted | 100 | 167 | 32 | 25 | 22 | 20 | 17 |
| Banana<br>1 med. | 150 | 127 | 24 | 19 | 17 | 15 | 13 |
| Blackberries, raw<br>1 cup | 144 | 84 | 16 | 13 | 11 | 10 | 8 |
| Blackberries, canned<br>1/2 cup, juice pack | 115 | 62 | 12 | 9 | 8 | 7 | 6 |
| Blueberries, raw<br>5/8 cup | 100 | 62 | 12 | 10 | 8 | 7 | 6 |
| Boysenberries, frozen without sugar<br>4/5 cup | 100 | 48 | 9 | 7 | 6 | 6 | 5 |
| Cantaloupe, raw<br>1/4 melon, 5″ diam. | 100 | 30 | 6 | 4 | 4 | 4 | 3 |
| Cherries, sweet, raw<br>24 small, 15 large | 100 | 70 | 14 | 10 | 9 | 8 | 7 |
| Cherries, sweet, canned<br>1/2 cup, water pack | 100 | 43 | 8 | 6 | 6 | 5 | 4 |
| Cranberry sauce<br>5 tbs. (rounded) | 100 | 146 | 28 | 22 | 19 | 17 | 15 |
| Fruit cocktail<br>1/2 cup, water pack | 100 | 37 | 7 | 6 | 5 | 4 | 4 |
| Fruit cocktail, heavy syrup<br>1/2 cup | 100 | 76 | 14 | 12 | 10 | 9 | 8 |
| Grapefruit, raw<br>1/2 medium | 100 | 40 | 8 | 6 | 5 | 5 | 4 |
| Grapes, American<br>22 medium | 100 | 70 | 14 | 10 | 9 | 8 | 7 |
| Guava, raw<br>1 medium | 100 | 62 | 12 | 9 | 8 | 7 | 6 |

## Exercise Equivalents of Food Calories in Minutes

### Table 11 (cont.)

| FOOD | WEIGHT 1oz.=30gm | CALORIES | WALKING | BICYCLING | STEPPING | SWIMMING | JOGGING |
|------|------|------|------|------|------|------|------|
| | gm. | kcal. | min. | min. | min. | min. | min. |
| Honeydew, raw 1/4 small (5" diam.) | 100 | 33 | 6 | 5 | 4 | 4 | 3 |
| Lemon, raw 1/4 medium | 25 | 7 | 1 | 1 | 1 | 1 | 1 |
| Lychees, raw 3 1/2 oz. | 100 | 64 | 12 | 10 | 9 | 8 | 6 |
| Mango, raw 1/2 medium | 100 | 66 | 13 | 10 | 9 | 8 | 7 |
| Nectarine, raw 1 medium | 50 | 32 | 6 | 5 | 4 | 4 | 3 |
| Olives, green, packed 4 medium | 26 | 30 | 6 | 4 | 4 | 4 | 3 |
| Olives, ripe 4 large | 40 | 74 | 14 | 11 | 10 | 9 | 7 |
| Orange, raw 1 medium (3" diam.) | 150 | 73 | 14 | 11 | 10 | 9 | 7 |
| Papaya, raw 1/2 medium | 165 | 65 | 13 | 10 | 9 | 8 | 7 |
| Peaches, raw 1 medium | 100 | 38 | 7 | 6 | 5 | 4 | 4 |
| Peaches, canned, heavy syrup 2 med. halves | 100 | 78 | 15 | 12 | 10 | 9 | 8 |
| Peaches, canned, juice pack 2 halves | 100 | 45 | 9 | 7 | 6 | 5 | 5 |
| Pears, raw 1 medium | 200 | 122 | 24 | 18 | 16 | 14 | 12 |
| Pears, canned, water pack 2/5 cup | 100 | 32 | 6 | 5 | 4 | 4 | 3 |
| Persimmons, raw 1 medium | 100 | 77 | 15 | 12 | 10 | 9 | 8 |
| Pineapple, raw 1 slice (3 1/2" × 3/4") | 84 | 44 | 9 | 7 | 6 | 5 | 4 |

46

Table 11 (cont.)

| FOOD | WEIGHT 1oz.=30gm | CALORIES | WALKING | BICYCLING | STEPPING | SWIMMING | JOGGING |
|---|---|---|---|---|---|---|---|
| | gm. | kcal. | min. | min. | min. | min. | min. |
| Pineapple, canned, heavy syrup 1 large slice | 100 | 74 | 14 | 11 | 10 | 9 | 7 |
| Pineapple, canned, juice pack 1 large slice | 100 | 58 | 11 | 9 | 8 | 7 | 6 |
| Plums, raw 2 medium | 100 | 66 | 13 | 10 | 9 | 8 | 7 |
| Prunes, dry 8 large | 100 | 344 | 66 | 52 | 46 | 41 | 34 |
| Prunes, dry, cooked (no sugar) 5 med.; 2 tbs. juice | 100 | 120 | 23 | 18 | 16 | 14 | 12 |
| Raisins, dried 1 tbs. | 10 | 30 | 6 | 4 | 4 | 4 | 3 |
| Raspberries, raw, black 2/3 cup | 100 | 75 | 14 | 11 | 10 | 9 | 8 |
| Strawberries, raw 10 large | 100 | 37 | 7 | 6 | 5 | 4 | 4 |
| Strawberries, frozen, with sugar 1/2 cup | 128 | 140 | 27 | 22 | 19 | 17 | 14 |
| Strawberries with cream, sugar 10 large; 4 tbs.; 2 tsp. | 170 | 197 | 38 | 30 | 26 | 24 | 20 |
| Tangerine, raw 1 large | 100 | 46 | 9 | 7 | 6 | 6 | 5 |
| Watermelon, raw 1 wedge (4″ × 8″) | 925 | 115 | 22 | 17 | 15 | 14 | 12 |
| FRUIT JUICES | | | | | | | |
| Apple juice, fresh 1/2 glass (4 oz.) | 120 | 60 | 12 | 9 | 8 | 7 | 6 |

# Exercise Equivalents of Food Calories in Minutes

## Table 11 (cont.)

| FOOD | WEIGHT 1oz.=30gm gm. | CALORIES kcal. | WALKING min. | BICYCLING min. | STEPPING min. | SWIMMING min. | JOGGING min. |
|---|---|---|---|---|---|---|---|
| Apricot juice <br> ½ glass (4 oz.) | 120 | 60 | 12 | 9 | 8 | 7 | 6 |
| Cranberry juice cocktail <br> ½ glass (4 oz.) | 120 | 82 | 16 | 13 | 11 | 10 | 8 |
| Cranberry-apple juice <br> ½ glass (4 oz.) | 120 | 80 | 15 | 12 | 11 | 10 | 8 |
| Grapefruit juice <br> ½ glass (4 oz.) | 120 | 47 | 9 | 7 | 6 | 6 | 5 |
| Grape juice <br> ½ glass (4 oz.) | 120 | 80 | 15 | 12 | 11 | 10 | 8 |
| Lemonade <br> 1 glass (8 oz.) | 240 | 105 | 20 | 16 | 14 | 13 | 11 |
| Orange juice <br> ½ glass (4 oz.) | 120 | 54 | 10 | 8 | 7 | 6 | 5 |
| Papaya juice <br> ½ glass (4 oz.) | 120 | 60 | 12 | 9 | 8 | 7 | 6 |
| Punch, Hawaiian <br> ½ glass (4 oz.) | 120 | 108 | 21 | 17 | 14 | 13 | 11 |
| Prune juice <br> ½ glass (4 oz.) | 120 | 92 | 18 | 14 | 12 | 11 | 9 |
| Tomato juice <br> ½ glass (4 oz.) | 120 | 23 | 4 | 3 | 3 | 3 | 2 |
| Vegetable juice, canned <br> ½ glass (4 oz.) | 120 | 21 | 4 | 3 | 3 | 3 | 2 |
| **MEATS** | | | | | | | |
| Bacon, crisp fried <br> 2 strips (20 strips/lb) | 15 | 90 | 17 | 14 | 12 | 11 | 9 |
| Beef: | | | | | | | |
| Club steak, broiled <br> 3 oz. cooked | 90 | 175 | 33 | 26 | 23 | 21 | 18 |

# Table 11 (cont.)

| FOOD | WEIGHT 1oz.=30gm | CALORIES | WALKING | BICYCLING | STEPPING | SWIMMING | JOGGING |
|---|---|---|---|---|---|---|---|
| | gm. | kcal. | min. | min. | min. | min. | min. |
| Corned beef, canned<br>2 slices (3″ × 2″ × ¼″) | 56 | 120 | 23 | 18 | 16 | 14 | 12 |
| Hamburger, cooked<br>1 patty (3″ diam. × 1″) | 85 | 224 | 43 | 34 | 30 | 27 | 22 |
| Porterhouse, broiled<br>3 oz. cooked | 90 | 175 | 33 | 26 | 23 | 21 | 18 |
| Pot roast, lean only<br>3 oz., cooked | 90 | 168 | 32 | 26 | 22 | 20 | 17 |
| Rib roast<br>2 slices (4″ × 2½″ × ½″) | 105 | 240 | 46 | 36 | 31 | 29 | 24 |
| Round, broiled<br>1 slice (4″ × 3″ × 1″) | 120 | 218 | 41 | 33 | 28 | 26 | 22 |
| Rump roast<br>2 slices (4″ × 1¼″ × ½″) | 90 | 165 | 31 | 25 | 21 | 20 | 17 |
| Short ribs, broiled<br>1 serving (3 oz. cooked) | 90 | 220 | 42 | 33 | 29 | 26 | 22 |
| Sirloin steak, broiled<br>3 oz. cooked | 90 | 175 | 33 | 26 | 23 | 21 | 18 |
| T-bone steak, broiled<br>3 oz. cooked | 90 | 175 | 33 | 26 | 23 | 21 | 18 |
| Tenderloin, broiled<br>3 oz. cooked | 90 | 175 | 33 | 26 | 23 | 21 | 18 |
| Beef & vegetable stew<br>1 cup | 235 | 210 | 40 | 31 | 27 | 25 | 21 |
| Chili con carne with beans<br>1 cup | 250 | 334 | 64 | 50 | 44 | 40 | 33 |
| Chili con carne, no beans<br>1 cup | 250 | 358 | 68 | 55 | 48 | 43 | 36 |
| Frankfurter (weiner)<br>1 frank (8/lb pkg.) | 56 | 170 | 32 | 26 | 22 | 20 | 17 |
| Ham, fresh, cooked<br>2 slices (3 oz. cooked) | 90 | 254 | 49 | 38 | 34 | 30 | 25 |

# Exercise Equivalents of Food Calories in Minutes

**Table 11 (cont.)**

| FOOD | WEIGHT 1oz.=30gm gm. | CALORIES kcal. | WALKING min. | BICYCLING min. | STEPPING min. | SWIMMING min. | JOGGING min. |
|---|---|---|---|---|---|---|---|
| Lamb chop<br>2 chops (3 oz. cooked) | 90 | 205 | 39 | 31 | 27 | 25 | 21 |
| Lamb, roast<br>2 slices (4″ × 3″ × 1/4″) | 90 | 192 | 37 | 29 | 26 | 23 | 19 |
| Liver, beef or pork<br>2 slices (3″ × 2¼″ × 3/8″) | 75 | 170 | 33 | 26 | 23 | 20 | 17 |
| Meat loaf, beef<br>1 slice (4″ × 3″ × 3/8″) | 70 | 140 | 27 | 22 | 19 | 17 | 14 |
| Meat loaf, beef and pork<br>1 slice (4″ × 3″ × 3/8″) | 70 | 264 | 51 | 40 | 35 | 32 | 26 |
| Pork chops, lean<br>2 chops (3 oz. cooked) | 90 | 260 | 49 | 39 | 34 | 31 | 26 |
| Pork roast<br>3 slices (2½″ × 1″ × ½″) | 70 | 160 | 31 | 24 | 21 | 19 | 16 |
| Pork, spareribs<br>6 med. ribs (3 oz. uncooked) | 90 | 246 | 47 | 37 | 33 | 30 | 25 |
| Rabbit, baked<br>3 oz. | 90 | 160 | 30 | 25 | 21 | 19 | 16 |
| Raccoon, baked<br>3 oz. | 90 | 230 | 44 | 35 | 31 | 28 | 23 |
| Sausage—see under<br>  Sausages | | | | | | | |
| Veal, roast, lean only<br>3 oz. | 90 | 136 | 26 | 21 | 18 | 16 | 14 |
| Venison, fresh, cooked<br>3 oz. | 90 | 180 | 34 | 28 | 24 | 22 | 18 |
| NUTS | | | | | | | |
| Almonds, chocolate<br>10 med. | 28 | 142 | 27 | 21 | 19 | 17 | 14 |

Table 11 (cont.)

| FOOD | WEIGHT 1oz=30gm gm. | CALORIES kcal. | WALKING min. | BICYCLING min. | STEPPING min. | SWIMMING min. | JOGGING min. |
|---|---|---|---|---|---|---|---|
| Almonds, dried, salted 12–15 nuts | 15 | 93 | 18 | 14 | 12 | 11 | 9 |
| Brazil nuts, shelled 4 med. | 15 | 97 | 19 | 15 | 13 | 12 | 10 |
| Cashew nuts, roasted 6–8 nuts | 15 | 84 | 16 | 13 | 11 | 10 | 8 |
| Coconut, shredded, dried 2 tbsp. | 15 | 83 | 16 | 12 | 11 | 10 | 8 |
| Hazel (filberts) nuts 10–12 nuts | 15 | 97 | 19 | 15 | 13 | 12 | 10 |
| Macadamia nuts 6 whole | 15 | 110 | 21 | 16 | 15 | 13 | 11 |
| Mixed nuts 8–12 nuts | 15 | 94 | 18 | 14 | 13 | 11 | 9 |
| Mixed nuts, dry roasted 10–12 nuts | 15 | 85 | 16 | 13 | 11 | 10 | 8 |
| Peanuts, dry roasted 8–10 nuts | 16 | 80 | 15 | 12 | 11 | 10 | 8 |
| Peanuts, roasted 6–8 nuts | 15 | 86 | 17 | 13 | 11 | 10 | 9 |
| Pecans 12 halves | 15 | 104 | 20 | 16 | 14 | 12 | 10 |
| Pinyon nuts 2 tbs. | 15 | 95 | 18 | 14 | 13 | 11 | 10 |
| Pistachios 30 nuts | 15 | 88 | 17 | 13 | 12 | 11 | 9 |
| Soybeans, dry, cooked 20–25 beans | 15 | 20 | 4 | 3 | 3 | 2 | 2 |
| Sunflower Seeds 30–40 nuts | 15 | 84 | 16 | 13 | 11 | 10 | 8 |
| Walnuts 8–10 halves | 15 | 94 | 18 | 14 | 13 | 11 | 9 |

# Exercise Equivalents of Food Calories in Minutes

**Table 11 (cont.)**

| FOOD | WEIGHT 1oz.=30gm | CALORIES | WALKING | BICYCLING | STEPPING | SWIMMING | JOGGING |
|---|---|---|---|---|---|---|---|
| | gm. | kcal. | min. | min. | min. | min. | min. |
| POULTRY | | | | | | | |
| Chicken, breast, broiled 1/2 breast (no bone) | 72 | 105 | 20 | 16 | 14 | 13 | 11 |
| Chicken, breast, fried 1/2 breast (no bone) | 76 | 155 | 29 | 23 | 20 | 19 | 16 |
| Chicken, leg, broiled 1 med. (no bone) | 35 | 52 | 10 | 8 | 7 | 6 | 5 |
| Chicken, leg, fried 1 med. (no bone) | 38 | 90 | 17 | 14 | 12 | 11 | 9 |
| Chicken, wing, broiled 2 med. (no bone) | 35 | 90 | 17 | 14 | 12 | 11 | 9 |
| Chicken, wing, fried 2 med. (no bone) | 38 | 126 | 24 | 19 | 17 | 15 | 13 |
| Chicken, roasted 2 slices (3" × 3" × 1/4") | 80 | 158 | 30 | 24 | 21 | 19 | 16 |
| Chicken, roasted with gravy 2 slices; 2 tbs. | 115 | 238 | 46 | 36 | 32 | 29 | 24 |
| Duck, roasted 2 slices (3 1/2" × 2 1/2" × 1/4") | 70 | 218 | 42 | 33 | 29 | 26 | 22 |
| Turkey, roasted 2 slices (3" × 3" × 1/4") | 80 | 160 | 31 | 24 | 21 | 19 | 16 |
| Turkey, roasted with gravy 2 slices; 2 tbs. | 115 | 240 | 46 | 36 | 32 | 29 | 24 |
| SALADS AND SALAD DRESSING | | | | | | | |
| Apple, celery, walnuts with mayonnaise 1 serving; 1 tbsp. | 168 | 237 | 46 | 36 | 32 | 28 | 24 |
| Chicken with celery 3 tbsp.; 2 leaves lettuce | 146 | 185 | 35 | 28 | 25 | 22 | 19 |

# Table 11 (cont.)

| FOOD | WEIGHT 1oz.=30gm | CALORIES | WALKING | BICYCLING | STEPPING | SWIMMING | JOGGING |
|---|---|---|---|---|---|---|---|
| | gm. | kcal. | min. | min. | min. | min. | min. |
| Apricots, cottage cheese<br>3 med. halves; 2 tbs. | 156 | 98 | 19 | 15 | 13 | 12 | 10 |
| Coleslaw<br>2/3 cup | 84 | 68 | 13 | 10 | 9 | 8 | 7 |
| Fruit mixture<br>3 tbs.; 2 lettuce leaves | 193 | 155 | 30 | 23 | 21 | 19 | 16 |
| Gelatin with fruit, on lettuce<br>1 square, (3″ × 3″ × 1″) | 188 | 140 | 27 | 21 | 19 | 17 | 14 |
| Lettuce, french dressing<br>1 wedge; 2 tbs. | 130 | 133 | 26 | 20 | 18 | 16 | 13 |
| Lettuce, tomato, mayonnaise<br>4 leaves; 3 slices; 1 tsp. | 115 | 80 | 15 | 12 | 11 | 10 | 8 |
| Peach with cottage cheese<br>2 med. halves; 2 tbs.<br>  cheese | 156 | 105 | 20 | 16 | 14 | 13 | 10 |
| Potato salad<br>1/2 cup | 100 | 99 | 19 | 15 | 13 | 12 | 10 |
| Tomato, tuna salad<br>1 med.; 2 tbs. | 180 | 100 | 19 | 15 | 13 | 12 | 10 |
| Salad dressings (1 tbs.): | | | | | | | |
| Blue cheese (Roquefort) | 14 | 70 | 14 | 10 | 9 | 8 | 7 |
| Low calorie* | 14 | 15 | 3 | 2 | 2 | 2 | 1 |
| French dressing | 14 | 57 | 11 | 9 | 8 | 7 | 6 |
| Italian dressing | 14 | 77 | 15 | 12 | 10 | 9 | 8 |
| Mayonnaise | 14 | 100 | 19 | 15 | 13 | 12 | 10 |
| Tartar sauce | 14 | 75 | 14 | 11 | 10 | 9 | 8 |
| Thousand island | 14 | 80 | 15 | 12 | 10 | 10 | 8 |

*The calorie content of various brands and types will vary.

# Exercise Equivalents of Food Calories in Minutes

## Table 11 (cont.)

| FOOD | WEIGHT 1oz.=30gm | CALORIES | WALKING | BICYCLING | STEPPING | SWIMMING | JOGGING |
|---|---|---|---|---|---|---|---|
| | gm. | kcal. | min. | min. | min. | min. | min. |
| **SANDWICHES †** | | | | | | | |
| Bacon, lettuce, tomato 1, white, toasted | 148 | 282 | 54 | 42 | 38 | 34 | 28 |
| Bologna with mayonnaise 1 slice; 1 tsp. | 68 | 220 | 42 | 33 | 29 | 26 | 22 |
| Cheese, toasted | 85 | 286 | 55 | 43 | 38 | 34 | 29 |
| Cheese, fried egg, lettuce 1 slice; 1 egg, 1 leaf | 135 | 344 | 66 | 52 | 46 | 41 | 34 |
| Cheeseburger | 180 | 462 | 89 | 69 | 61 | 55 | 46 |
| Chicken, hot, with gravy 3 tbsp. gravy | 160 | 356 | 69 | 53 | 47 | 43 | 36 |
| Chicken, with mayonnaise 2 slices (3″ × 3″ × ¼″) | 126 | 310 | 59 | 48 | 41 | 37 | 31 |
| Chicken salad | 110 | 245 | 47 | 37 | 33 | 29 | 25 |
| Club (bacon, chicken, tomato) 3 slices toast, lettuce | 315 | 590 | 114 | 88 | 78 | 71 | 59 |
| Corned beef | 102 | 240 | 46 | 37 | 32 | 29 | 24 |
| Egg salad | 138 | 280 | 54 | 42 | 37 | 34 | 28 |
| Fried egg | 100 | 222 | 43 | 33 | 30 | 27 | 22 |
| Ham | 81 | 280 | 54 | 42 | 38 | 34 | 28 |
| Ham and cheese 1 slice; 1 slice | 111 | 390 | 74 | 60 | 52 | 47 | 39 |
| Hamburger | 150 | 350 | 57 | 52 | 47 | 42 | 35 |
| Ham salad | 114 | 320 | 62 | 48 | 43 | 38 | 32 |
| Hot dog with ketchup | 110 | 258 | 50 | 39 | 34 | 31 | 26 |

†Two slices of bread for all sandwiches unless specified otherwise.

## Table 11 (cont.)

| FOOD | WEIGHT 1oz.–30gm | CALORIES | WALKING | BICYCLING | STEPPING | SWIMMING | JOGGING |
|---|---|---|---|---|---|---|---|
| | gm. | kcal. | min. | min. | min. | min. | min. |
| Jelly, assorted | 43 | 115 | 22 | 18 | 15 | 14 | 12 |
| Liverwurst | 91 | 250 | 48 | 38 | 33 | 30 | 25 |
| Peanut butter | 83 | 328 | 63 | 49 | 44 | 39 | 33 |
| Peanut butter and jelly 1 rd tbs.; 1 level tbs. | 86 | 290 | 55 | 45 | 39 | 35 | 29 |
| Roast beef, lettuce, mayonnaise | 125 | 400 | 77 | 60 | 63 | 48 | 40 |
| Roast beef, hot with gravy | 160 | 430 | 83 | 64 | 57 | 52 | 43 |
| Roast pork, hot with gravy 3 tbs. gravy | 180 | 503 | 97 | 75 | 67 | 60 | 50 |
| Roast pork, lettuce with mayonnaise | 125 | 470 | 90 | 70 | 63 | 56 | 47 |
| Salami with mayonnaise 1 slice; 1 tsp. | 80 | 283 | 54 | 44 | 38 | 34 | 28 |
| Tuna fish salad | 105 | 278 | 54 | 42 | 37 | 33 | 28 |
| Turkey, cold with mayonnaise 1 tsp. mayonnaise | 125 | 284 | 55 | 43 | 38 | 34 | 28 |
| Turkey, hot with gravy 3 tbsp. gravy | 156 | 402 | 77 | 60 | 53 | 48 | 40 |
| SAUCES * | | | | | | | |
| Barbecue, hot ¼ cup | 50 | 60 | 11 | 9 | 8 | 7 | 6 |
| Cheese, sauce 2 tbsp | 38 | 65 | 12 | 10 | 9 | 8 | 7 |

*Vegetables cooked without oil or butter except as specified.

# Exercise Equivalents of Food Calories in Minutes

## Table 11 (cont.)

| FOOD | WEIGHT 1oz.=30gm | CALORIES | WALKING | BICYCLING | STEPPING | SWIMMING | JOGGING |
|---|---|---|---|---|---|---|---|
| | gm. | kcal. | min. | min. | min. | min. | min. |
| Chili sauce<br>1 tbsp | 17 | 17 | 3 | 3 | 2 | 2 | 2 |
| Cocktail sauce<br>1 tbsp | 15 | 25 | 5 | 4 | 3 | 3 | 3 |
| Horseradish<br>1 tbsp | 15 | 16 | 3 | 2 | 2 | 2 | 2 |
| Meat sauce<br>1 tbsp | 15 | 20 | 4 | 3 | 3 | 2 | 2 |
| Mustard, yellow<br>1 tbsp | 15 | 11 | 2 | 2 | 1 | 1 | 1 |
| Sour cream sauce<br>1/4 cup | 50 | 140 | 27 | 22 | 19 | 17 | 14 |
| Soy sauce<br>1 tbsp | 15 | 8 | 2 | 1 | 1 | 1 | 1 |
| Steak sauce<br>1 tbsp | 15 | 10 | 2 | 2 | 1 | 1 | 1 |
| Worcestershire sauce | 15 | 12 | 2 | 2 | 2 | 1 | 1 |
| **SAUSAGES** | | | | | | | |
| Beef and pork, link<br>1 link (2 1/4" × 1 1/2" diam) | 60 | 252 | 49 | 38 | 34 | 30 | 25 |
| Bologna<br>1 slice (4 1/2" diam × 1/8") | 30 | 66 | 13 | 10 | 9 | 8 | 7 |
| Frankfurter<br>1 ave. (8/lb pkg.) | 56 | 170 | 32 | 26 | 22 | 20 | 17 |
| Liver sausage<br>1 slice (3" diam. × 1/4") | 30 | 80 | 15 | 12 | 11 | 10 | 8 |
| Luncheon meat<br>1 slice (4 1/2" diam. × 1/4") | 30 | 80 | 15 | 12 | 11 | 10 | 8 |

# Table 11 (cont.)

| FOOD | WEIGHT 1oz.=30gm gm. | CALORIES kcal. | WALKING min. | BICYCLING min. | STEPPING min. | SWIMMING min. | JOGGING min. |
|---|---|---|---|---|---|---|---|
| Pork sausage 1 patty, 2″ diam. | 22 | 100 | 19 | 15 | 13 | 12 | 10 |
| Pork sausage 1 link (3″ × ½″) | 20 | 94 | 18 | 14 | 13 | 11 | 9 |
| Salami 1 slice 3¾″ × ¼″) | 30 | 130 | 25 | 20 | 17 | 16 | 13 |
| Vienna sausage 1 ave. (2″ × ¾″) | 18 | 40 | 8 | 6 | 5 | 5 | 4 |
| SEA FOODS—FISH | | | | | | | |
| Abalone, canned 3½ oz. | 100 | 80 | 15 | 12 | 11 | 10 | 8 |
| Anchovy, canned 3 thin fillets | 12 | 20 | 4 | 3 | 3 | 2 | 2 |
| Anchovy paste 1 tsp. | 7 | 14 | 3 | 2 | 2 | 2 | 1 |
| Bass, baked 1 serving (3″ × 3″ × ½″) | 115 | 287 | 55 | 43 | 38 | 34 | 29 |
| Carp, fried 3½ oz.; 1 tbs. oil | 100 | 280 | 53 | 42 | 35 | 34 | 28 |
| Catfish, fried 3½ oz.; 1 tbs. oil | 100 | 270 | 51 | 40 | 35 | 32 | 27 |
| Caviar, canned 1 rd. tsp. | 10 | 32 | 6 | 5 | 4 | 4 | 3 |
| Clams 5 large or 10 small | 100 | 80 | 15 | 12 | 11 | 10 | 8 |
| Cod, broiled 3 oz. | 90 | 162 | 31 | 24 | 22 | 19 | 16 |
| Crab, steamed 3½ oz. | 100 | 93 | 18 | 14 | 12 | 11 | 9 |

# Exercise Equivalents of Food Calories in Minutes

## Table 11 (cont.)

| FOOD | WEIGHT 1oz.=30gm | CALORIES | WALKING | BICYCLING | STEPPING | SWIMMING | JOGGING |
|---|---|---|---|---|---|---|---|
| | gm. | kcal. | min. | min. | min. | min. | min. |
| Flounder or sole, baked 1 serving | 100 | 202 | 38 | 31 | 27 | 24 | 20 |
| Frog legs, fried 3 large legs | 72 | 210 | 40 | 32 | 28 | 25 | 21 |
| Haddock, fried 1 fillet (3" × 3" × ½") | 100 | 165 | 31 | 25 | 22 | 20 | 17 |
| Halibut, broiled 4 oz. | 120 | 214 | 41 | 32 | 28 | 26 | 21 |
| Herring, pickled 3½ oz. | 100 | 223 | 43 | 33 | 30 | 27 | 22 |
| Lobster, boiled with butter 1; 2 tbs. butter | 334 | 308 | 59 | 46 | 41 | 37 | 31 |
| Lobster Newburg 6½ oz. | 195 | 377 | 72 | 58 | 50 | 45 | 38 |
| Mackerel, broiled 1 fillet (4½ oz.) | 130 | 300 | 58 | 45 | 40 | 36 | 30 |
| Mackerel, canned ½ cup | 105 | 192 | 36 | 30 | 26 | 23 | 19 |
| Oysters, raw 5–8 medium | 100 | 66 | 13 | 10 | 9 | 8 | 7 |
| Perch, fried 1 serving | 65 | 108 | 21 | 16 | 14 | 13 | 11 |
| Pike, Northern, raw 3½ oz. | 100 | 88 | 17 | 14 | 12 | 11 | 9 |
| Salmon, baked 3½ oz. | 100 | 182 | 35 | 27 | 24 | 22 | 18 |
| Salmon, pink, canned ⅖ cup | 100 | 141 | 27 | 22 | 19 | 17 | 14 |
| Sardines, Canned in Oil 8 medium | 100 | 311 | 59 | 48 | 41 | 37 | 31 |
| Sardines in tomato sauce 1½ large | 100 | 197 | 38 | 30 | 26 | 24 | 20 |

# Table 11 (cont.)

| FOOD | WEIGHT 1oz.=30gm | CALORIES | WALKING | BICYCLING | STEPPING | SWIMMING | JOGGING |
|---|---|---|---|---|---|---|---|
| | gm. | kcal. | min. | min. | min. | min. | min. |
| Scallops, fried, breaded 3½ oz. | 100 | 194 | 37 | 29 | 26 | 23 | 19 |
| Sea bass, raw 3½ oz. | 100 | 96 | 19 | 14 | 13 | 12 | 10 |
| Shrimp, French fried 3½ oz. | 100 | 225 | 43 | 34 | 30 | 27 | 23 |
| Trout, brook, raw 3½ oz. | 100 | 100 | 19 | 15 | 13 | 12 | 10 |
| Trout, lake (under 6 lbs. raw) 3½ oz. | 100 | 240 | 46 | 36 | 32 | 29 | 24 |
| Tuna, canned in oil, drained 3 oz. | 90 | 170 | 32 | 26 | 22 | 20 | 17 |
| Tuna, canned in water ½ cup | 100 | 127 | 24 | 20 | 17 | 15 | 13 |
| Tuna and noodle casserole 4 oz. | 120 | 192 | 36 | 30 | 26 | 23 | 19 |
| SOUPS—1 cup | | | | | | | |
| Bean with pork | 250 | 170 | 33 | 26 | 23 | 20 | 17 |
| Beef broth | 240 | 30 | 6 | 5 | 4 | 4 | 3 |
| Beef noodle | 240 | 70 | 14 | 10 | 9 | 8 | 7 |
| Bouillon | 240 | 8 | 2 | 1 | 1 | 1 | 1 |
| Chicken noodle | 240 | 62 | 12 | 10 | 8 | 7 | 6 |
| Clam chowder, Manhattan | 240 | 80 | 15 | 12 | 10 | 10 | 8 |
| Clam chowder, New England | 240 | 150 | 28 | 23 | 20 | 18 | 15 |
| Cream of celery | 240 | 120 | 23 | 18 | 16 | 14 | 12 |

# Exercise Equivalents of Food Calories in Minutes

## Table 11 (cont.)

| FOOD | WEIGHT 1oz.=30gm gm. | CALORIES kcal. | WALKING min. | BICYCLING min. | STEPPING min. | SWIMMING min. | JOGGING min. |
|---|---|---|---|---|---|---|---|
| Cream of chicken, with milk | 240 | 180 | 35 | 27 | 24 | 22 | 18 |
| Cream of mushroom, with milk | 240 | 215 | 41 | 32 | 29 | 26 | 22 |
| Cream of tomato | 240 | 165 | 31 | 25 | 22 | 20 | 17 |
| Minestrone | 245 | 105 | 20 | 16 | 14 | 13 | 11 |
| Onion | 240 | 38 | 7 | 6 | 5 | 5 | 4 |
| Oyster stew | 240 | 200 | 39 | 30 | 27 | 24 | 20 |
| Split pea | 245 | 145 | 28 | 22 | 19 | 17 | 15 |
| Tomato | 245 | 90 | 17 | 14 | 12 | 11 | 9 |
| Vegetable | 240 | 77 | 15 | 12 | 10 | 9 | 8 |
| Vegetable beef | 245 | 90 | 15 | 12 | 11 | 10 | 8 |
| | | | | | | | |
| TV DINNERS (COMPLETE) | | | | | | | |
| Beef TV dinner | 310 | 350 | 67 | 52 | 47 | 42 | 35 |
| Beef meat pie | 230 | 445 | 86 | 67 | 59 | 53 | 46 |
| Chicken meat pie | 230 | 505 | 97 | 76 | 67 | 61 | 51 |
| Chicken TV dinner, fried | 310 | 542 | 104 | 81 | 72 | 65 | 54 |
| Chopped sirloin TV dinner | 270 | 485 | 93 | 73 | 65 | 58 | 49 |
| Haddock TV dinner | 340 | 328 | 63 | 49 | 44 | 39 | 33 |
| Ham TV dinner | 285 | 310 | 60 | 46 | 41 | 37 | 31 |
| Loin of pork TV dinner | 285 | 414 | 80 | 62 | 55 | 50 | 41 |
| Meat loaf TV dinner | 310 | 370 | 71 | 56 | 49 | 44 | 37 |
| Pizza, cheese 1/8 of 14″ diam. pie | 75 | 185 | 36 | 28 | 25 | 22 | 19 |
| Pizza, sausage 1/8 of 14″ diam. pie | 75 | 195 | 38 | 29 | 26 | 23 | 20 |

# Table 11 (cont.)

| FOOD | WEIGHT 1oz.=30gm | CALORIES | WALKING | BICYCLING | STEPPING | SWIMMING | JOGGING |
|---|---|---|---|---|---|---|---|
| | gm. | kcal. | min. | min. | min. | min. | min. |
| Swiss steak TV dinner | 285 | 250 | 48 | 38 | 33 | 30 | 25 |
| Turkey meat pie | 230 | 420 | 81 | 63 | 56 | 50 | 42 |
| **VEGETABLES \*** | | | | | | | |
| Asparagus, cooked 4 spears | 60 | 10 | 2 | 2 | 1 | 1 | 1 |
| Asparagus with mayonnaise 4 spears; 1 tsp. | 65 | 44 | 9 | 7 | 6 | 5 | 4 |
| Beans, baked (molasses sauce) ½ cup | 125 | 142 | 27 | 22 | 19 | 17 | 14 |
| Beans, lima ½ cup | 85 | 95 | 18 | 14 | 13 | 11 | 10 |
| Beans, snap, green ½ cup | 62 | 15 | 3 | 2 | 2 | 2 | 2 |
| Bean sprouts 1 cup | 100 | 28 | 5 | 4 | 4 | 3 | 3 |
| Beans with pork and tomato ½ cup | 125 | 152 | 29 | 23 | 20 | 18 | 15 |
| Beans with pork and molasses ½ cup | 125 | 188 | 36 | 28 | 25 | 23 | 19 |
| Beets, red, diced ½ cup | 83 | 27 | 5 | 4 | 4 | 3 | 3 |
| Beet greens, cooked ½ cup | 100 | 18 | 4 | 3 | 2 | 2 | 2 |
| Broccoli 1 stalk, 5½" | 100 | 32 | 6 | 5 | 4 | 4 | 3 |

\*Most spices and herbs add virtually no calories in the quantities used.

# Exercise Equivalents of Food Calories in Minutes

## Table 11 (cont.)

| FOOD | WEIGHT 1oz.=30gm gm. | CALORIES kcal. | WALKING min. | BICYCLING min. | STEPPING min. | SWIMMING min. | JOGGING min. |
|---|---|---|---|---|---|---|---|
| Brussels sprouts $^2/_3$ cup | 100 | 36 | 7 | 5 | 5 | 4 | 4 |
| Cabbage, cooked 1 cup | 145 | 30 | 6 | 5 | 4 | 4 | 3 |
| Cabbage, raw, shredded 1 cup | 90 | 20 | 4 | 3 | 3 | 2 | 2 |
| Cabbage with coleslaw dressing 1 cup; 1 tbs. | 90 | 126 | 24 | 19 | 17 | 15 | 13 |
| Carrots, cooked, drained $^2/_3$ cup | 100 | 31 | 6 | 5 | 4 | 4 | 3 |
| Carrots, raw 1 large or 2 small | 100 | 42 | 8 | 6 | 6 | 5 | 4 |
| Cauliflower, cooked, drained $^7/_8$ cup | 100 | 31 | 6 | 5 | 4 | 4 | 3 |
| Cauliflower, raw, with mayonnaise 1 cup; 1 tsp. | 105 | 60 | 12 | 9 | 8 | 7 | 6 |
| Celery 2 small stalks (5") | 40 | 6 | 1 | 1 | 1 | 1 | 1 |
| Collards, cooked 1 cup | 190 | 55 | 11 | 8 | 7 | 7 | 6 |
| Corn, sweet 1 ear | 140 | 70 | 14 | 10 | 9 | 8 | 7 |
| Corn, sweet, buttered 1 ear; 1 tsp. | 145 | 105 | 20 | 16 | 14 | 13 | 11 |
| Corn, sweet, canned $^1/_2$ cup | 128 | 85 | 16 | 13 | 11 | 10 | 9 |
| Corn, sweet, cream style $^1/_2$ cup | 100 | 85 | 16 | 13 | 11 | 10 | 9 |
| Cowpeas, cooked $^1/_2$ cup | 80 | 86 | 17 | 13 | 11 | 10 | 9 |

# Table 11 (cont.)

| FOOD | WEIGHT 1oz.=30gm gm. | CALORIES kcal. | WALKING min. | BICYCLING min. | STEPPING min. | SWIMMING min. | JOGGING min. |
|---|---|---|---|---|---|---|---|
| Cucumber, raw<br>6 slices, 1/8″ | 50 | 5 | 1 | 1 | 1 | 1 | 1 |
| Eggplant, cooked<br>1/2 cup | 100 | 19 | 4 | 3 | 3 | 2 | 2 |
| Lettuce, cos, romaine<br>3 1/2 oz. | 100 | 18 | 3 | 3 | 2 | 2 | 2 |
| Lettuce, iceberg<br>1/8 head (4 3/4″ diam) | 55 | 10 | 2 | 2 | 1 | 1 | 1 |
| Lettuce with salad dressing<br>1/8 head; 1 tbsp. | 70 | 70 | 14 | 10 | 9 | 8 | 7 |
| Mushrooms, canned<br>1/2 cup | 100 | 17 | 3 | 3 | 2 | 2 | 2 |
| Mushrooms, fresh, raw<br>10 small or 4 large | 100 | 28 | 5 | 4 | 4 | 3 | 3 |
| Mushrooms, fried<br>4 med. | 70 | 78 | 15 | 12 | 10 | 9 | 8 |
| Onions, cooked<br>1/2 cup | 105 | 30 | 6 | 4 | 4 | 4 | 3 |
| Onions, raw<br>1/2 onion (2 1/2″ diam) | 55 | 20 | 4 | 3 | 3 | 2 | 2 |
| Peas, green, cooked<br>1/2 cup | 80 | 58 | 11 | 9 | 8 | 7 | 6 |
| Peppers, green<br>1 large, empty shell | 100 | 22 | 4 | 3 | 3 | 3 | 2 |
| Peppers, stuffed<br>1 large; grd. beef | 185 | 246 | 47 | 37 | 33 | 30 | 25 |
| Pickles, dill<br>1 med. | 65 | 10 | 2 | 2 | 1 | 1 | 1 |
| Pickles, sweet<br>1 large | 100 | 146 | 28 | 22 | 19 | 18 | 15 |
| Poi, two-finger<br>1 cup | 250 | 166 | 32 | 25 | 22 | 20 | 17 |

# Exercise Equivalents of Food Calories in Minutes

## Table 11 (cont.)

| FOOD | WEIGHT 1oz.=30gm gm. | CALORIES kcal. | WALKING min. | BICYCLING min. | STEPPING min. | SWIMMING min. | JOGGING min. |
|---|---|---|---|---|---|---|---|
| Potato, baked 1 med. | 99 | 90 | 17 | 14 | 12 | 11 | 9 |
| Potato, baked with butter 1 med.; 2 pats | 110 | 160 | 31 | 24 | 21 | 19 | 16 |
| Potato, baked with sour cream 1 med.; 2 tbs. | 130 | 140 | 27 | 21 | 19 | 17 | 14 |
| Potato chips 10 pieces (2″ diam) | 20 | 115 | 22 | 17 | 15 | 14 | 12 |
| Potatoes, french fries 20 pieces (½″ × ½″ × 2″) | 100 | 274 | 53 | 41 | 36 | 33 | 27 |
| Potatoes, hashed brown ½ cup | 100 | 230 | 44 | 34 | 31 | 28 | 23 |
| Potatoes, mashed (with milk and butter) ½ cup | 100 | 94 | 18 | 14 | 13 | 11 | 9 |
| Potatoes, mashed with gravy ½ cup; 2 tbsp. | 136 | 174 | 34 | 26 | 23 | 21 | 17 |
| Radishes, red, raw 5 small | 50 | 8 | 1 | 1 | 1 | 1 | 1 |
| Sauerkraut, canned ½ cup | 115 | 22 | 4 | 3 | 3 | 3 | 2 |
| Sauerkraut with weiners ½ cup; 1 weiner | 170 | 146 | 28 | 22 | 19 | 18 | 15 |
| Soybean curd (tofu) 3½ oz. | 100 | 72 | 14 | 11 | 10 | 9 | 7 |
| Spinach, Cooked ½ cup | 90 | 20 | 4 | 3 | 3 | 2 | 2 |
| Spinach, raw 3½ oz. | 100 | 26 | 5 | 4 | 3 | 3 | 3 |

# Table 11 (cont.)

| FOOD | WEIGHT 1oz.=30gm gm. | CALORIES kcal. | WALKING min. | BICYCLING min. | STEPPING min. | SWIMMING min. | JOGGING min. |
|---|---|---|---|---|---|---|---|
| Squash, summer, cooked ½ cup | 105 | 14 | 3 | 2 | 2 | 2 | 1 |
| Squash, winter, baked ½ cup | 100 | 63 | 12 | 10 | 8 | 8 | 6 |
| Sweet potatoes, baked 1 small | 100 | 140 | 27 | 21 | 19 | 17 | 14 |
| Sweet potatoes, candied 2 halves | 100 | 168 | 32 | 25 | 22 | 20 | 17 |
| Tomato, cooked ½ cup | 100 | 26 | 5 | 4 | 3 | 3 | 3 |
| Tomato, raw 1 med (3" diam) | 200 | 40 | 8 | 6 | 5 | 5 | 4 |
| Tomato catsup 1 tbsp. | 17 | 18 | 4 | 3 | 2 | 2 | 2 |
| Turnip greens, cooked 1 cup | 145 | 30 | 6 | 4 | 4 | 4 | 3 |
| Turnips, cooked ½ cup | 75 | 18 | 4 | 3 | 2 | 2 | 2 |

# Notes

1. F. Konishi, "Food Energy Equivalents of Various Activities," *J. Am. Diet Assoc.* 46 (1965): 186.

2. M. L. Hathaway and E. D. Foard, *Heights and Weights of Adults in the United States*, Home Economics Research Report No. 10 (Washington, D.C.: U.S. Department of Agriculture, 1960).

3. National Research Council, *Recommended Dietary Allowances*, 7th ed., National Academy of Sciences, Publication 1694 (Washington, D.C., 1968).

4. A. Keys and F. Grande, "Body Weight, Body Composition, and Calorie Status," in *Modern Nutrition in Health and Disease*, by M. G. Wohl and R. S. Goodhart, 4th ed. (Philadelphia, 1968).

5. National Research Council, *Recommended Dietary Allowances*.

6. J. E. Brockett, F. Konishi et al., *The Energy Expenditure of Soldiers in a Training Company*, USAMNL Report No. 212, 1957; R. Passmore and J. V. G. A. Durnin, "Human Energy Expenditure," *Phsiol. Rev.* 35 (1955): 801.

7. Passmore and Durnin, p. 801.

8. Brockett, Konishi et al.; Passmore and Durnin, p. 801; E. M. Widdowson et al., "The Food Intake and Energy Expenditure of Cadets in Training," *Brit. J. Nutrition* 8 (1954): 147.

# Index

69

# Index

# Index

# Index

# Index

# Index

# Index